AN ORGASMIC CONNECTION TO AN EVER CHANGING UNIVERSE

AN ORGASMIC CONNECTION TO AN EVER CHANGING UNIVERSE

◆

A handbook for personal/planetary survival, and pleasure, for the next century

Dr. Robert W. Kessel DSW LCSW BCD

iUniverse, Inc.

New York Lincoln Shanghai

AN ORGASMIC CONNECTION TO AN EVER CHANGING UNIVERSE
A handbook for personal/planetary survival, and pleasure, for the next century

iUniverse books may be ordered through booksellers or by contacting:

iUniverse
2021 Pine Lake Road, Suite 100
Lincoln, NE 68512
www.iuniverse.com
1-800-Authors (1-800-288-4677)

ISBN-13: 978-0-595-37934-7 (pbk)
ISBN-13: 978-0-595-82304-8 (ebk)
ISBN-10: 0-595-37934-6 (pbk)
ISBN-10: 0-595-82304-1 (ebk)

Printed in the United States of America

Contents

A brief review.

Thoughts and ideas can leave an emotional legacy for future generations.

An adventure of discovery, to explore new ideas and ways to map your reality; and to increase skills as a traveler.

The journey of life depends upon where you travel, and how you are as a traveler.

There are not just laws embedded in the universe waiting to be discovered; there are agreements waiting to be made.

We embark upon an orgasmic connection to an ever changing universe.

ACKNOWLEDGEMENTS

One of the principles enunciated in this book is that of a universal <u>connection</u> to everything and everyone both in the past, and present; the writing of this book reflects this basic idea. Any accomplishment is accompanied by a large measure of shared credit, (and hopefully not blame). The source of my ideas are many and varied, and I admit to a feeble attempt in expressing my gratitude as well as begging your forgiveness for my many omissions. I begin by offering my heart felt thanks and appreciation to the following: To my many gurus, masters,and teachers who graciously offered their knowledge, wisdom and guidance < I hold you close to my heart and celebrate my contacts and memories of our moments. To my family and early friends affording the common mixture of pain and love, both necessary for growth, I offer much appreciation and love for their support and sustenance. To "Big John" Lykes, who has recently left this planet, I miss your sharing of your photographic memory covering a wide range of topics, never a boring moment, To Todd Cleary and Nahtahna Cabanes for their supportive editing advice, and for putting up with my endless chatter about my book. To Noel and Kat Blanc, two highly talented individuals who provided much appreciated support and suggestions for my effort as well as valuable advice from their own successful careers. To John and JoAnn Braheny a very gifted duo sharing their business experience in writing and publishing in the field of music, adding their voices to the chorus of support. To my neighbor Wes and Corey Hanson, he for his insightful and creative suggestions, she for her quiet support. To Donna Fisher a fellow spiritual traveler, for her helpful editing and suggestions. To Susan Casey who while writing her own book took the time to provide me with many helpful suggestions and encouragement, (and her book was published). To Cindy Mcquade who provided ongoing, enthusiastic support, encouragement, and a good ear for my occasional rants, and to David Mayhan for his contribution to the glossary. To Jorge Almeida who provided a much enthusiastic and encouraging reception of an early reading of sections of my book. To Dr. Noah McKay who inspired his audience relating his own life changing experience at a recent conference. To Issac Cohen who has offered his service to promote the book to other parts of the world. To Eric Weinstein with his knowledge and ability with computers kept me reasonably sane as I tried to negotiate in that somewhat hostile environment, and to Katarina Ericksson who with her gentle manner calmed my lion nature when the chips were down in my computer universe. A special thanks to Kristina Andresen who took time out from her very busy schedule as an architect to lay out the format for creating a reader friendly document. Finally, to an unknown source that energized, motivated and inspired me to finally write our manuscript. We all share in this book.

Dr Bob

INTRODUCTION

I invite you to join me in a journey of exploration that offers opportunities for personal change and growth, empowering you to deal with the complex, and frequently baffling issues that face citizens of the 21st century. Like most journeys one must prepare, opening the door for a holistic approach to life, combing our mind, body, and spirit as one synergistic and cohesive unit; providing the means to a deeper understanding of ourselves as well as the issues we face in the 21st century.

You begin a conscious journey of not knowing who you are.

We live in an age of Accelerating Acceleration wherein changes at the micro and macro level of human experience are proceeding at an exponential level. We note rapid changes in technology, communication, commerce, and political/economic areas that are dramatically impinging upon people's wellbeing and life style. It is the magnitude of change, which effects more and more people, giving rise to the sense that the earth is shrinking, that people are impacting each other with greater force and frequency.

In order to deal with the changes of the 21st century <u>we</u> must be the most significant change.

We can no longer hide behind our wall of oceans. Our borders are no longer secure and the idea of a unified nation/state is fading, as the rise of powerful corporations grow beyond national boundaries and create new allegiances with vague accountability. The nation/state may evolve into the corporate/state forming a new entity with uncertain qualities of governance. The one critical change that is yet to happen in a significant and rapid fashion is personal growth and enlightenment; a necessity in order to better appreciate and develop a more sensitive understanding of our dramatically changing modern world. It has been said that the pace of discovery and change that occurred in the 20th century, will occur in just a 20 year period in the 21st century. Yet while our species has the greatest impact upon the planet, we seem to be much slower in our own development, and ability to manage and effectively cope with this accelerated pace of change.

The purpose of this book is to suggest new ways of viewing the world and suggest creative ways of "thinking" about who we are, as we shape our experience of the world. The choices we make as well as the motivations behind these choices will not only effect our lives but the lives of future generations as well as the wellbeing of the planet. With this purpose in mind, we will revisit old arguments about how we know what we know; why we remain fixed in our views and belief systems; and how we can improve our understanding and awareness of the dynamic changes in our personal, social, political, and ultimately spiritual lifestyles. At a personal level our own health and wellbeing is at stake. We cannot limit our understanding of health as simply the absence of disease, but we must broaden our understanding of health to include all of life, including the wellbeing of the planet, which is not separate from who we are. Health can no longer be separated by mind and body (the result of a historical argument between a French philosopher and the Catholic Church in the 17 th century). In order to confront and deal with the changes of the 21st century we must be the most significant change. To this end, this book is dedicated.

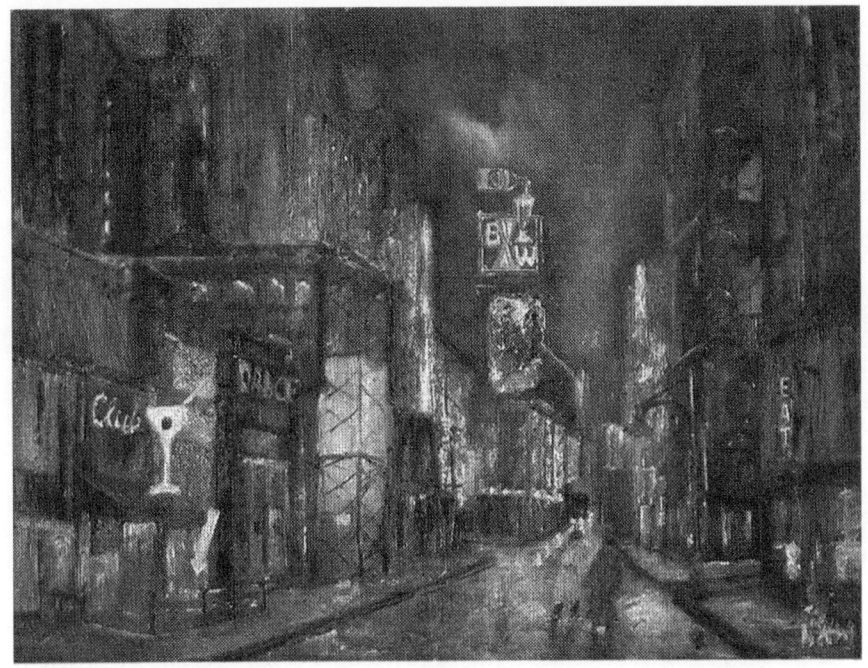

Art by Norman W Merrill

The closer you come to the horizon of knowing the further it retreats

INITIAL JOURNEY PREPARATIONS

To begin our preparations we must revisit a historic argument that has been a foundation and cornerstone for western thought. In his book Zen and the Art of Motorcycle Maintenance the author Robert Persig, a professor in a college in Montana examines the nature and quality of explanation, (what ever else they do, professors are involved in explaining things, examining ideas, and doing research so as to continue to teach and explain new ideas and so forth and so on). The basic question is how does one evaluate the quality of various explanations. To examine this fundamental issue, Professor Persig returns to ancient Greece, the birth place of western philosophy to examine a basic disagreement between two philosophical perspectives as represented by two groups: the Aristotelians and the Sophists. The Aristotelians believed that the value of explanation is fundamentally related to whether the explanation was true. Explanations which were not true were of no value. In our culture we continuously search out the truth and nothing but the truth. It is our legal oath and it's also written in the halls of our many universities. Truth has historically been the basis for our science although lately we have been hearing about probability theory (probably true? What's that?) The Sophists on the other hand felt that the value of explanation had more to do with the effects of the explanation upon the human condition. Did the explanation raise the spiritual, creative levels, offer opportunities for human growth and development, and in some way benefit human kind.

Consider the excluded middle.

These were two historical positions, Aristotelian having to do with the right or wrong, true or false, valid or invalid. There was no middle ground. One always searched for the final or ultimate principle. Sophists emphasized the effects of the explanation upon the human condition. Negative effects demeaning the human condition preventing growth and development were of less value; positive effects enhancing the human condition were desired. Persig notes that at this important juncture of western thought Aristotelian ideas prevailed and became the foundation of western thinking. Persig ends his exploration of the value of explanation with a question. What if the wrong side won the argument? If the wrong side won, then the basis of western thought would rest upon a faulty premise.

No one knows the whole story of an unfolding one.

After much thought (as a former professor what am I supposed to do but reflect and think) the question raised by Persig is an Aristotelian question; the "wrong" side versus the "right" side is an "either/or" question and maintains the Aristotelian search for "truth".

Certainty aborts the journey of discovery.

In order to prepare for our journey, we must heal this historical argument and recognize the value of both positions, neither of which is the whole story. The notion that truth carries with it certainty, accuracy, preciseness, and completeness has changed. In science we see the advent of probability theory and chaos theory that raise the uncertainty level of the ideas we consider truthful. The accuracy and certainty of truth can most often be found in our models and in our symbolic representations of reality, which are not the reality itself. The axiom that "the map is not the territory" reminds us of this inexact fit. Nevertheless, certain accepted truths can be useful such as found in mathematics or in certain sciences. In today's world of the sophisticated and widespread use of mass media and other opinion and belief influencing technologies; we must approach the bits of truth with a mind set of the impact of the truth on the human condition. Specifically, who and what does the truth serve? Does the truth excite our negative emotions such as fear or anger? Does the truth have some self-serving purpose on the part of the source? Does the information resonate with our deeper understanding and intuitive awareness? Does the information harmonize with our "gut feeling" and "body wisdom"? Are we emotionally open and sufficiently detached to truly "understand" with a mind/body consideration, or are we looking for belief systems under the guise of information to confirm our own strongly held beliefs and opinions? When we are open and emotionally in balance, we can consider the "information value" of various ideas, combining our sense of truth and the quality of spiritual integrity to enhance the human condition. Often this will be a better judgment than a simple true or false position.

The map is not the territory.

Very often, in language, words have hidden meaning. The word "understand" is one such word. That word consists of two words: under and stand. If you were to transpose these words you would create the word "stand under" which directs one to go beneath that which is being communicated. To truly understand one must lower his/her response time to feel and reflect with both the heart and mind and consider with a deeper and intuitive consideration. All of this requires time and delay. Typical communication is much faster. Each person in a conversation awaits a psychological "green light"; impatient for the pause and communication space so as to offer their opinion and prove whatever he/she has to prove which typically is, how intelligent, how well-informed, how knowledgeable, and how personally adequate one is, as well as being right. Taking time to consider and reflect can frequently provide a much more powerful response, especially if it is a heartfelt intuitive response raising the likelihood of an <u>epiphamonious</u> experience for the speaker. Allowing sufficient time to reflect and consider raises the opportunity for a mind/body period of incubation leading to a more developed response. This offers a deeper understanding for the listener. The speaker is encouraged by reflective support to explore his inner wisdom while the listener benefits from a more thoughtful and wiser answer.

In a conversation, waiting for a green light is a sign of heavy traffic.

THE "EPIPHAMONIOUS" JOURNEY

The word epiphany has several meanings including religious contacts with holy figures as well as a manifestations of a deity. The word also describes "a sudden, intuitive perception or insight into the reality or essential meaning of something."

"Standing under" a conversation often leads to a "heart felt response".

Central to the meaning of this word is A SUDDEN POWERFUL AWAKENING to a richer, deeper fuller awareness and appreciation of a fundamental meaning that resonates with one's heart/mind, body, and spirit. At times it has been described as the "aha" response, an experience of sudden insight. As part of this journey I, as the facilitator, will use various variations of this word in different forms, as a noun, modifier, and perhaps even as a verb, none of which will likely be found in the dictionary. As part of the adventure, you dear reader, will need to navigate the meaning. However, not to despair; for various ideas and thoughts will be offered as tools to equip you as an "Epiphamonious" adventurer on a journey toward multiple epiphanies. (a sense of humor will often ease any journey)

Knowledge is learned, wisdom is discovered.

As part of this search for deeper meaning and resounding under-standing, we need to be reminded of a number of adages that have a ring of epiphamonious truth. Two such sayings derive from historical esoteric knowledge. They are: You begin a conscious journey of not knowing who you are, and secondly, the closer you come to the horizon of knowing, the further it retreats. Both of these sayings remind us of the uncertainty of knowing, as well as the changing nature of knowledge. To this is added the modern day mantra of; *no one knows the whole story*. With these ideas as travel markers we begin to discern important features in the landscape which are pitfalls to avoid. There are several. The first being; beware of premature knowledge closure. Certainty aborts the journey of discovery and impedes our evolutionary process. Certainty, when it fills our sense of knowing, eliminates the growth of ideas, and dulls the mind to change and new discovery. Related to that pitfall is "either/or" thinking which denies any value to the other side so that your side is the only right one. This is not to say that one cannot hold a contrary opinion but rather to underscore the idea that not every discussion is a debate to be won, (often a hidden power struggle to prove personal competence).

When one supports the integrity and ability of others to embark upon their own evolutionary journey, in harmony with the interconnectedness of the whole, that is moral behavior.

Another pitfall to avoid is premature epistemological consciousness closure. Epistemology is an area of study that deals with a fundamental question of how do we know what we know. What is the basis for our ideas, beliefs, and information. This approach to information underscores the basis of our culture and history. One can argue that the great strides in western civilization came about during times of conceptual revolutions or epistemological shifts. For example; prior to the development of Greek Philosophy with its emphasis on reason and deductive logic, supernatural explanation and story telling were primary ways of developing an information and cultural belief system. Greek Philosophy provided a reasoned, although flawed, order to the universe. Centuries later the Copernican Revolution (named after an obscure Polish mathematician) gave rise to an approach to knowledge using an inductive form of logic based upon observation and measurement. Thus began the birth of classical science and the resulting development of navigation, leading to national exploration and expansion. New forms of mechanical advancement led to developments in transportation and mechanization which fueled the the beginnings of the Industrial Revolution. National Power shifted away from those societies that did not make this conceptual shift (usually based upon religious dogma);to those nations that developed the technology based upon this new paradigm. Along with this new shift was a deterministic belief that the universes worked as a great machine based upon basic laws embedded in nature, and that these laws could be discovered by careful observation and measurement. Thus the idea that given a camera that could take enough accurate pictures of the universe; everything that could be known will be known; thereby giving rise to the image of man positioned outside of nature, controlling the universe through the emergence of his new science and technology; an idea that still lingers to this day.

Certainty, when it fills our sense of knowing, eliminates the growth of ideas, and dulls the mind to change and new discovery.

We also note an acceleration of these conceptual shifts. More than twenty centuries passed between the ancient Greek approach to knowledge to the birth of Classical Science. More recent conceptual shifts have occurred in a shorter time span. Advances made in the science of physics and astronomy created a mind staggering view of the universe. These developments along with the discovery of the vastness and complexity of subatomic space created the next conceptual shift into what some have called the Age of Relativity. While attempts to adhere to scientific principles remained, it was now understood that the observer influenced the observed. In other words, there was no fixed or unchanging camera to take objective pictures of the universe. Scientific findings and results reflected the attributes of the technologies used to find those results.

WHAT IS TECHNOLOGY BUT AN EXTENSION OF HUMAN CONSCIOUSNESS

In a relatively short period of time other epistemological shifts have occurred which have dramatically impacted upon the *"gathering-of-knowledge"* landscape. Very recent changes include a more inclusive way of *"knowing"*, no longer limited to the intellect. With the rise of parapsychology, and an increasing interest in metaphysical studies, information and ideas are being generated that are no longer constrained by rigorous guidelines of scientific validation or intellectual study. Trance states, (e.g. Edger Cayce), channeling, and other esoteric abilities are being used. The wide spread use of mind altering substances has opened up other avenues in the search for *"truth"*. The most current shift is based upon the coming together of western materialism, and eastern philosophy and mysticism, the result of increasing cultural contact and exchange. As a result, spiritual matters are increasingly matters of concern reflecting the greater interest in non-materialism of many non-western cultures. Recent explorations and developments in the science of physics having to do with the advent of quantum physics and string theory confound much of our rationally accepted beliefs as well as (in the case of string theory} our foundation of logic. Lastly, studies in the area of Synchronicty wherein human cells, human cycles, as well as machines, appear to significantly influence each other based upon close proximity [e.g. heart cells in separate petri dishes, close to each other, synchronize beats] hold a promise of new forms of healing through the transmission of energy and communication which has yet to be fully understood. New research in Nanotechnology (miniaturization to the atomic level) may effect how we effect changes at a level previously unthinkable, as we enter a new universe of opportunity and discovery. One significant conclusion stands out from all of these conceptual shifts; a never-ending story can not be the whole story. We must open ourselves to the possibilities which cannot be seen or perhaps even imagined. When we think we know the answer, the journey stops.

Life can be lived as an adventure to be explored or as a problem to be avoided

SOCIAL AND CULTURAL CEMENT

Fundamental to any culture is the way that culture deals with change. History is the accounting and explanation of cultural change. Various cultures can be examined as to whether new ideas, inventions, or changing demographics, are accepted, resisted, or altered. This provides a measure of the capacity of a culture to adapt and evolve to changing condition while maintaining the quality of cultural life. On a more personal level, change can be examined from the perspective of an individual trying to cope with any number of personal challenges as they deal with their life within the context of that culture, Every individual has a road map or belief system related to the nature of change both in relation to a personal as well as a cultural level. Whether its a discussion of national politics, economics, or ones' personal life there is an implied or a clearly stated model of change. That model sets the parameters for change thereby promoting greater freedom and opportunity or restricting the potential for creative change.

Armed with an increasing skill of epiphamonious travel we are becoming better prepared to journey forth. We continue preparing for our journey by examining a fundamental principle in western thought and western science which has to do with the nature of change. It's called the "Cause and Effect model of change." Something happens which creates or causes a specific result. In medicine we look for the magic bullet to cure a particular disease. In history we look for specific events that created significant historical changes. Our models of explanation in the biological sciences, economics, and until recently, physics were heavily underpinned with this model. We have been looking for specific causes to explain specific outcomes. In the behavioral sciences we argued over whether it was heredity vs. environment, nature vs. nurture, and genes vs. lifestyle (the same argument with different words) that are the ultimate determinants of who we are, how we live, and how we maintain our health and wellbeing. Often these arguments were colored by the arrogance of experts to show the "rightness" of their position and the "wrongness" of their opponents. {Arrogance is defined as denying the experience, beliefs and ideas of others and offering ones own as the only true explanation.} (Expert is defined as someone who appears less uncertain than the rest of us.} Inherent in that model is the idea that an active agent acts upon a passive agent causing changes in the latter. Be it a drug "curing" a disease, a product improving our life, or an historical event causing dramatic significant changes in history, there is a specific cause identified. In advertising and marketing the Cause/Effect model is used to sell specialized products, or unique change agents to create personal financial, social, and sexual success, so that there is a financial interest in supporting that model of change. In the world of dogmatic ideas, ideology, and entrenched views of history and nature, that model abounds.

The Cause/Effect model is an overly simplified explanation of change leading to theoretical camps that combat and compete over their views and beliefs. <u>The conflict is inherent in the nature of the model itself and not always in the differing views.</u> Thus we have different groups explaining health and wellness issues, political and economic issues, and religious and spiritual issues in certain and fixed way so as to exclude other points of view. Remember, nothing is the whole story and history has repeatedly shown that such groups rigidly intolerant and fixed in the certainty of their beliefs have most often been the greatest road blocks toward evolutionary progress and understanding. Dogma, when it seeks to explain the whole story, limits further awareness and aborts one's epiphamonious journey.

One does not create a road map for unexplored territory'.

THE AGE OF ACCELERATING ACCELERATION

What gives the impression of "new" is the acceleration of the "old."

In order to consider a new model for explaining change, we have to appreciate a basic premise which is increasingly obvious in the 21st century. We live in an age of accelerating information, ideas, and increased social contact help create a shrinking world wherein events in one part of the globe quickly effect other parts. The pace of change has increased in tempo and in scope. Human impact upon the planet is more dramatic and significant. We can no longer deny our collective impact upon the earth and each other. Given the rise of complexity and uncertainty, a simple Cause/Effect model of change, which may be better suited to a controlled environment such as a laboratory, is less useful to explain social phenomena. The idea of a single causative factor is less likely to be accepted in todays world of probability theory and the emerging uncertainty of chaos theory. What is more likely to be observed (with careful scrutiny) is that certain tendencies exist, and some event or stimulus occurs, which causes an abrupt acceleration of those same tendencies, giving the impression of a new development. As an example, a car driving over a nail results in a flat tire. Most people would say that the nail caused the tire to go flat. Focus is placed upon the nail as the cause and the tire is ignored as a dynamic force. In an acceleration model of change, the dynamic features of the tire are considered. The tire is seen as containing air pressure which seeks to escape the confines of the tire. We all recognize the need to monitor air pressure as needed due to the loss of air. The nail punctures the tire and accelerates a direction or tendency that already exists and it is this complex interaction between a tendency and an accelerant that brings about the observed change. The tire is not a passive object or recipient of an outside force that is the total cause for change. An acceleration model of change offers a fuller understanding of the complex dynamics of change which reflect a complex field of various competing and interacting forces For example, we can no longer accept simple answers such as Hitler created Nazi Germany; or Sadaam Hussein was the creator of the tyranny in Iraq. In science such thinking is labeled as the "Pitfall of Reductionism" i.e. reducing complex data which covers various disciplines to one discipline offering one answer. We can also appreciate that many new discoveries and findings are not new, rather they are an acceleration of present factors which suddenly receive wider recognition giving rise to a sense of new discovery.

We live in a world of accelerating acceleration which effects our sense of spiritual balance.

Creative change and ideas are already "out there" waiting for a mind that is tuned to their existence, able to pull these ideas into conscious awareness. This is often the experience of discovery described by innovative thinkers, and remember, this is not the whole story of discovery.

THE PITFALL OF MACRO AND MICRO ANALYSIS

To change an uncaring bureaucracy, we must create bureaucrats that care.

The social and behavioral sciences are separated by the size of the phenomena studied. Micro sciences study smaller sized populations such as individuals, small groups and family groups. Larger populations such as cultural and societal groups as well as a variety of social institutions including historical development are the subjects for Macro analysis. This separation and compartmentalizing for study purposes limits the development of strategies for change at the macro levels; for it is only individuals that can change. We often assign human characteristics to inanimate concepts such as compassionate conservative, a hostile culture, a depressed or anxious social class, etc. We talk as if these human qualities actually exist in non-human form apart from human beings. In order to effect changes and development in areas where human qualities have been assigned to abstract concepts we have to influence people. For it is only people that can express compassion, make fair-minded decisions and act in a caring fashion. There is a pressing need to develop effective strategies to enhance and encourage life enhancing decisions, policies, and programs on the part of people who staff our social and political institutions: to change an uncaring bureaucracy to bureaucrats that care.

Much of media news consists of having a biased source feeding a belief system under the guise of information to the preconceived notions of various groups of people.

Strategies for change already exist within the form of mass media as well as the field of education. But too often the true purpose of providing unbiased information is subverted by the source to influence people rather than to educate them. Much of our current news reporting tells stories to persuade people rather than to inform them. Most people choose stories that confirm an already held position or belief thus they support the current news reporting situation. News organizations motivated by money, the so called "bottom line" (the holy grail of business) provide a sellable product rather than a factual one. In a sense we are returning to the ancient past wherein communication was primarily oral in nature, using storytelling, fables and parables which were designed to influence people as well as maintain a cultural/religious tradition. The notion of accurate reporting was not part of a cultural mentality since much explanation was predetermined by past religious and cultural stories. Investigative journalism was for the most part not yet developed. The problem persists of having a biased source feeding a belief system under the guise of information to the preconceived notions of various groups of people. This contributes to much distortion and lack of understanding on topics and issues which increasingly impact greater numbers of people. This is a recipe for disaster in the 21st century. We have to formulate a better road map to prepare for our journey of not knowing who we are, not knowing the whole story of an unfolding story, and finally to find a good corn beef sandwich. (as well as deal with the planetary issues of the new century.) There is an old adage that; life can be lived as an adventure to be explored or as a problem to be avoided. Our epiphamonious journey takes the adventuresome path.

Much of our current news reporting tells stories to persuade people rather than to inform them.

THE PROBLEM OF "STICKYNESS"

Being Stuck (or BS, a shortened form) is a most significant factor in a number of human situations and is an impediment in our own personal journey. BS hinders personal growth, coping ability, problem solving skills, as well as ones spiritual evolution. We are all emotional beings experiencing a variety of fleeting and changing moods. We experience moments of joy, sadness, boredom, anger and a whole range of short and long term emotional states. These are part of the challenges and experience of being in our human bodies. It is when we become stuck in a given mind body/state such as an emotion or a belief which creates a problem for ourselves as well as others. For example, depression is not a problem. We all experience times and periods of feeling depressed. Periods vary depending, in part, on the experience trigger. Most often, we are able to move on to another experience of life resulting in changed feelings. It is when we become stuck in the feeling, when the feeling persists over time preventing our engagement with new experience and emotions; then we experience a problem of BS, not able to participate in the flow of life. The same is true for ideas and thinking although the pain felt may not be emotional in nature;nevertheless, BS in thinking and opinions can result in social consequences such as social isolation, boredom, limited association, repetitive conversations, and ignorance. Thus we ignore new ideas, changing conditions, and continue to navigate in denial (a river in the Mideast increasingly polluted by human contact, much like the politics of the region).

Traveling the highways of the mind can end up on never ending traffic circles.

When one is stuck in a past experience regardless whether its negative or positive; it keeps one stuck in the past. the greater the distance over time between that experience and the present is an indicator of an emotional disorder. Typically, many emotionally disturbed adults are stuck in past family problems which were experienced when they were a child. This BS impedes effective managing and coping of ones current reality. The problems of life continue to mount until one turns to drug use or serious mental/physical illness as a way of coping; living life as an increasingly burdensome problem.

Being "stuck" in our emotions and opinions prevents our engagement with new experiences and ideas, consequently less able to participate in the flow of life.

One of the greatest gifts parents can leave their children are good memories.

BS effects us in numerous and subtle ways, such as; body posture, facial configuration, diet, social contact, repetitive thoughts and addictive behavior. For example, at a physical level ones emotional state is reflected in posture, eye movement and the flexibility of facial muscles. Chronically depressed people typically slump, maintain their gaze below the horizon, and fix their facial muscles to complete an overall depressed look. One quick and simple remedy that illustrates the mind/body connection; there are approximately 45 facial muscles which are significantly connected to one's mood and emotional state. By altering the muscle tension and rearranging the facial look by a horizontal stretch of mouth and cheek muscles, commonly called a smile or grin; you can alter your mood, and also have the slight benefit of a facial skin treatment. You may also experience a feeling of being silly, which is a very good sign, For when you are feeling silly you are much less likely to feel depressed or any other negative emotion. In a sense you have taken an emotional vitamin which can be a significant remedy for negative emotional states, vitamin S or a silly pill. When you shift your gaze to above the horizon you are more likely to experience the feeling that things are looking up, life is looking better, however one can become less aware of stepping in dog droppings (an occasional side effect), Finally to complete this example; when one holds the body in a more upright position, eliminating the slump; one's connection to the world and flow of body energy will change, your emotions will improve, and people will respond in a positive way to your noticeable change in body language.

A significant remedy for negative emotions is vitamin S in the form of a "Silly Pill".

BS in your exercise regimen and patterns of movement exert a profound effect upon ones journey and overall health and wellbeing. One needs to vary exercise patterns to include cardiovascular, muscle strengthening, and range of motion stretches which will improve emotional and physical balance. The idea of exercise should be expanded to a more inclusive movement program which reflects your own evolution over time and relates to your mental, intuitive, and spiritual qualities. More will be said about this later.

Being caught in the mind dulls our other senses for zest full living.

As the human mind examines the observable universe one notes that all things develop in stages, whether they are inanimate or life forms. Stages in human development can be measured in a variety of ways including expected behavior for that stage; given the role of that person in a particular culture. For example, the expected behavior for a 3 year old child is different than a 21 year old adult. Each has a different position or status in the culture. BS is a significant factor in this area as well. The distance between social behavior and social status is an important measure of mental health and social functioning. If our 21 year old adult is acting like a 16 year old, we likely conclude that person is immature, If behavior is observed at a 3 year old level we see a severe emotional disorder. Being stuck or fixated at an earlier stage brings with it a range of mild, moderate, or severe dysfunction, both social and personal. One further note; many societies and cultures offer little if any behavioral expectations as people age beyond a certain stage. For example, In western society we often hear of a mid-life crisis as people move beyond the child rearing, homebuilding, success achieving, and "being pretty years". In this culture we are faced with uncertain expectations and confused direction for our creative "later years". So we often see older people continuing to act out the role expectations of an earlier stage creating BS in that earlier stage. We are also encouraged by manipulative and self-serving marketing to return to the behavior and values of an earlier stage. One health news letter offers you the secret thats "letting older men who were medical wrecks shape up instantly, surge with energy and steal the jobs and girlfriends of 30-year-olds." That is marketing BS of a different order.

The inner dialog or mental manuscript which deals with the injustices of the past, or the survival fears of the future, keeps us out of the fullness of the present.

A crucial part of BS relates to ones sense of personal identity. Too often in this and other industrial societies our sense of self is defined by,"who we are, is what we do." At a deeper, more spiritual level we rebel at this self defining notion. Once at an affair, in a circle of self introduction dominated by our work roles, this author added "who we are is not just what we do but rather who we are is what we drive". Of course, being in Malibu Ca. this was immediately accepted, and people added a description of the vehicles to their personal sense of identity.

A major determinant of our identity is the nature and the persistence of the questions we ask. Who we think we are determines to a very large extent the kinds of questions we raise. The nature of the questions can serve to keep us stuck, to narrow our vision, or to open new horizons to explore, and consequently, redefine ourselves and initiate a new journey. The questions we raise, serve to maintain our personal identity, often confused with "who we are".

We are like individual waves in a larger ocean, each wave is unique with its own particular qualities and direction that finally ends on a distant shore, yet all are part of the same ocean.

THE INNER DIALOGUE

There are any number of other major factors that both keep us predictable, set in our ways and views as well as impeding our spiritual awakening and epiphimonious journey. A number of years ago,this author composed an unwritten, unpublished manuscript entitled "Ortholinguistics, Healing the Inner Dialog". That mental manuscript dealt with the scientific fact that 99.846475% of our daily thoughts are repeats of yesterday's thoughts,and those thoughts followed repeated dramatic patterns or internal melodramas. Some common ones were,"Court Room". wherein one is preoccupied with proving oneself "right" while the other "wrong". One argues one's case in an imaginary court of law while being both judge and jury as well as the defense and prosecuting attorneys. The litigation never ends as long as one is caught up in the "injustices of the past". This is one of a variety of resentful anger and guilt issues anchored in the past which keeps us from experiencing the present. Another common mental scenario is "Survival of the Unfit", having to do with; who is going to care for me; how will I survive; a preoccupation with issues related to fear of the future. It is the never ending incessant internal chatter which serves as a psychological and emotional chain keeping us out of the fullness of the moment. Life then is experienced as a problem to avoid, rather than an unique adventure of the present.

Relationships and accounting don't add up.

From a mental health perspective, the inner dialog or inner conversation can range from a mild annoyance serving to distract or interfere with sleep, enjoyable sex, or an artistic moment, to more serious levels such as obsessive, intrusive, and delusional thinking, which can be symptoms of a serious mental disorder. In a sense, our inner upsetting thinking can be likened to an emotional fever, the greater the intensity and frequency, the greater the emotional upset. It is like "being caught in the mind", which dulls our other senses for zest full living. Persistent and reoccurring memories which are an important aspect of our inner dialogs can serve as a means to escape from an unpleasant present or as an anchor to a painful past. Either way, we are "captured" by the past significantly impacting our ability to live in the fullness of the moment and explore any adventuresome journey.

Reframing or changing assumptions and self imposed boundaries, increase opportunity, and greater personal control.

FILTERS and FRAMING

We all experience the world around us in different ways, and no two people experience the same event exactly in the same way. The idea of an "objective picture" of an experience or an event ignores the variety of differences among people who experience that event. At a purely physical level our five senses provide some information while eliminating other information. In other words we filter the experience taking in selected aspects while eliminating others; after all, that is the function of a filter to act as a screen. People's physical senses differ which in part explains different descriptions given for the same event. Just as we have sensory filters to order physical data, to keep from being overwhelmed by a barrage of sensory input; we also have filters to screen our thoughts and emotions. Filters serve to maintain our intellectual and emotional balance by maintaining our established beliefs and explanations. They provide a sense of order to our world and to our experience. Often filters support our emotional and intellectual positions by denying contrary information and accepting only confirming data. We seek confirmation from a variety of sources including friends, associates and the media. The rigidity of our filters are often a road block to any journey of personal growth including a greater understanding of our personal experience; as well as an effective role as a 21st century citizen, Emotional filters provide the glue, the passion, and the resistance to change, which anchors us to our beliefs. They form a significant portion of the core of our identity and keep us knowable and predictable to our friends and associates, who often also serve to maintain our views. Lest you think that filters are a deterrent to our journey, trapping you in analytical and experiential cement; take heart, we can evolve filters to aid our journey of personal growth. More will be said about that later.

Emotional, sensory, and intellectual filters act as a screen for human consciousness which maintain balance. Too restrictive, stunts growth, too fluid, creates confusion.

As we continue to prepare for our journey and move to more fully experience the moment, imagine, if you will, finding yourself enjoying a picture hanging on the wall, Notice the frame enclosing the picture. It contains all of the picture. Aha!! a possible insightful moment. Not unlike the picture frame, we also frame our experiences, resulting in our explanations and stories we tell ourselves and others, Often we are captured within our frames seeing no way out, limited by our self-imposed boundaries that tell "the whole story." The architecture of our framework, the lattice of our explanations offer an opportunity to climb out or be imprisoned in any given situation. Psychotherapist often use a technique of "reframing", helping the client to change the boundaries, assumptions, and self imposed limitations, thereby viewing the situation in a way which increase opportunity and greater control.

Filters can be evolved to aid our journey of personal growth.

The rigidity of our filters are most often a roadblock to any journey of personal growth, to greater understanding, and to an effective role as a 21st century citizen.

All of the above areas which have been briefly discussed; stickyness, the inner dialog, filters, and frames have other subtle and profound consequences for all of us. These elements exert profound effects upon the flow of energy within our bodies, the energy we radiate, and the nonverbal messages that are part of our unintended communication to others. The energy we transmit to others has many qualities among which are positive, negative and neutral effects. These energy forms carry with them healing, toxic, or neutral aspects for our own bodies as well as the those around us. These energy forms tend to be maintained over time unless conditions change. The basic principle is enunciated in the study of the field of Mind Science which is;"energy follows thought"; thinking negative thoughts creates negative energy within your body as well infecting those around you. We have all heard of a toxic relationships, toxic work environment, etc. The same principle holds true for positive and neutral energy which will effect our inner being and outer world. This will be explored further in an important section of our journey.

Energy follows thought, effecting you and those around you with positive, neutral, or negative energy.

THE LEGACY OF THE EXCLUDED MIDDLE

Think "yes and", rather than, "yes but", to create a fuller discussion, unless you really mean "yes but".

Life is not a debate to be won but an experience to be shared.

As mentioned in an earlier section of this book, western culture has opted for an Aristotelian form of explanation, searching for the "truth", rejecting the "non-true". This approach creates what is called the "excluded middle" there is no middle ground combing true/non-true existing together at the same time. What is generated in this method of either/or analysis is polar opposites, accepting one, rejecting the other, a frequently competitive exercise in the explanation discourse. What is essentially eliminated in this exclusion is a range of ideas offering a broader view, greater possibilities, and a cooperative spirit in the search for a reasoned explanation. A Hegelian model of the development of knowledge describes a discourse process of a thesis (statement}, an antithesis (a rebuttal), which than is incorporated into the original idea resulting in a more refined and better developed statement (synthesis). What is increasingly missing in todays political and cultural landscape is the coming together of ideas or the synthesis. Increasingly, the political view is, "your either with us or against us" The polar opposites remain at the poles giving rise to a new business of taking polls to measure the public support of polar positions. The middle ground is essentially frozen out of consideration. We have entered a new realm of "poll-land" in our search for answers. The media often supports the extremes by its attention and polling; further highlighting the seeming acceptance and importance of these positions. A recent example of this tendency toward divisiveness is the labeling of Republican states as "red" while the Democratic states are "blue" completely ignoring the mix of both parties as well as independent voters within all states. One can argue that the Blue and Red labels serve a political accounting purpose but as an acquaintance from Massachusetts reported, while visiting Florida, hearing one resident stating rather firmly that, "Florida was a Red state and that Kerry supporters were not welcome." The Blue and Red labels create a somewhat dramatic divide effecting an angry making separation of American citizens. A more extreme form could could create a Balkanizing effect renaming our country as The Divided States of America. The media is driven by ratings (read profit) and the need to increase their share of attention. The middle ground of discourse is less provoking less divisive and often lacks "shock value", supposably necessary for viewer attention. As a result, moderate views do not capture as much media expression as the extreme positions. In a culture of accelerating communication and the need for stimulation, a market is created for media content to meet these needs by focusing upon shock value programing, and inflammatory opinion.

Polar opposites create highly defined, restrictive perspectives than the larger more diffuse middle ground, which offers more personal choice.

Divide and conquer, unify and "hang out".

CONNECTION

Have you visited your molecular relatives floating in outer space?

From a spiritual perspective we acknowledge that everything in the universe shares a common connection from inner to outer space, from the macro to micro level, from animate to inanimate form, and to all planetary life and evolutionary development. We see evidence of this connection in new and startling ways. For example, we see galactic connections, as one galaxy appears to be "feeding" off of another by absorbing stars from the latter; a newly discovered "nursery", which appears to be a birth place for new stars and galaxies. These findings seem to reflect some of the conditions noted here on earth for creating and sustaining life. We have also observed our molecular relatives floating in outer space which are the same molecules that are part of our human bodies and physical heritage. Most importantly we note our personal connection to a universal presence which has had many different names and described in many different ways in human history. What than is this separation, this emphasis on difference, this ongoing polarity of either-or thinking? One source is the tendency to think in absolute terms violating the principle that no one knows the whole story; a fundamental precept to remain open and inclusive to ideas and experience. Our analytical minds also serve to separate ourselves from our experience by dividing data into segments for study and control purposes frequently losing the perspective of relationship and connection. The separation is in the mapping of the territory and not in the territory itself. By highlighting the parts, and thinking we can know the whole by the sum of its parts we return to a much earlier epistemological stage. In our current stage It is accepted that the universe opporates synergystically; that the whole is greater than the sum of its parts. It is these synergistic connections that need to be addressed, the subtle connections that serve to unify rather than divide, remembering that our need to divide carries with it the limitations of our senses, our limited observations, and imperfect methods of study. The 18th century idea of a perfect camera taking perfect pictures leading to a "perfect knowing" of the universe has been replaced by modern science's "probably so, but on the other hand."

We have a personal connection to a universal presence, which does not depend upon our financial support.

MINDBODY UNIFICATION

When it comes to personal health, lets all speak the same language.

As noted earlier the idea of separating mind from body occurred in the 17th century as part of a difference over turf control; the church maintaining control over the mind and soul of a person; the body given over to philosophy and medicine. Turf battles continue to this day with the difference being the arena of conflict. The separation of mindbody continues in our medical, social, and biological sciences each having staked out an area of specialized expertise related to a given part or "professional territory". Like most choices and agreements there have been gains and non gains, and in this age of accelerating acceleration there is enough information to "reshuffle the deck," and to "deal a new hand" to each of the scientific players. In a new game, new language and rules are required. The old game had language which only the insiders knew which was one of the advantages of membership. It served as a way maintaining boundaries and keeping the outsiders out. Citizenship in the 21st century requires at least an appreciation and general awareness of much of the knowledge base from which most people were formally excluded from in the 20th century. To this end, the language, concepts, and labels must have a descriptive quality of the phenomena it seeks to describe. Rather than using a dead language {Latin} or ancient melodramas (the Oedipal Conflict} The new language must be inclusive rather than exclusive; descriptive so that so that it is "user friendly." Ideas must not only be understood by the mind, but also felt by the soul [a bit of poetic license}. Increasingly, it is time for an informed knowledgeable consumer, using advice from an array of consultants and educators, to arrive at the best decisions; of particular importance in the field of healthcare.

Language, ideas, and intellect can serve to separate, divide, or unify, yielding profound consequences either way.

One idea that serves to end the conceptual separation of the mind from the body is the concept of a Psycho-Biological-Fabric or abbreviation PBF. We all have an image of a piece of cloth fabric. Now think of that fabric as a representation of the physical brain each interconnecting strand that compose that fabric is a bioenergetic transmission system that carries with it, a variety of social, psychological, family, and ultimately our personal life experience. How that is woven depends on the loom which we have inherited from our forebears. Some people have a sturdy loom, able to handle a variety of experiential threads, while others have more delicate weaving equipment, thus more sensitive to the thread of experience. Of course, that equipment can change over time, since its a dynamic entity and not just a piece of machinery (which is actually dynamic as well.) Since people have different experiences leading to varied and colorful patterns no two patterns are exactly the same. That fabric provides a substantial measure of who we are, how we think and feel, as well as behave. It is our personal and social identities comprising our beliefs, attitudes and values, forming the core of our experience on this planet. Many people would say, "that is who we are."

Oh what problems we weave with our Psycho/Biological Fabric.

The PBF is varied, dynamic and its actions can be measured in many different ways each giving a different picture as to the nature of that fabric depending upon the investigative approach. Returning to a previous incarnation of the PBF as simply being the brain, we can examine much of the scientific research. A biochemical approach yields a brain chemistry perspective, a landscape filled with a variety of neurotransmitters, neuropeptides, and other brain chemicals locking into an uptake or docking points located in specific portions of the brain in order to deliver various messages effecting our feelings and energy states. A "geographic mapping" of the brain leads to various sections of the brain, (lobes and hemispheres) with specialized functions as well as levels of functioning; lower order more primitive dealing with basic physical survival, to higher order dealing with rational thinking. A communication perspective highlights communication across a synapse or space to transmit nerve impulses to other other nerves, muscles or glands, a vast complex symphony keeping us in harmony with our environment. The brain also operates as an electrical system reflecting that investigative approach; certain areas "light up" in response to specific stimulation. Of course, none of this is the whole story as to how the brain functions. Recent research is highlighting specific responses of the brain to environmental stimulation underlying a basic connection of people to their environment. The notion of separation, the idea that people stand out side their environment separate from one another is rapidly fading. A recent article in the Los Angeles Times details the coming together of various disciplines in a rather ominous way. Scientists and "marketing professionals" are investigating consumer brain responses to specific stimuli for purposes of encouraging a brand loyalty to certain products; not unlike many politicians and political leaders who do much of the same.

Packaging is not more important than the product.

Separation is a figment of the mind.

PBF ADDICTION

Our explanations can serve to imprison or liberate others, as well as ourselves.

Probably the greatest impediment to growing and learning from one's life experience, is a Psycho-Biological-Fabric addiction which consist of being stuck or fixated in a variety of complex and interdependent ways. At a biological level, people become addicted to, and fixated upon, certain emotional states and feelings, both pleasant and unpleasant, This fixation includes a reoccurring electro-chemical pattern in the brain creating an attachment to that pattern not unlike other addictive drugs. In other words we assume a habitual repeating pattern of essentially the same brain chemistry and behavior with minor variations (reflecting the difference in daily experience). That repetition results in a cascade of fixations in our overall social and psychological functioning, including our emotional and energy state, behavioral patterns and habits, body posture, etc. At a psychological level the psychological/cognitive filters used to organize our views and perceptions of who we are, what we experience, and our explanations to ourselves and others, become rigid and fixed; an addiction to viewing and explaining our reality in a certain fixed way. This rigid acceptance of a given road map for navigating and reflecting upon our daily experience affords a sense of security in a world of uncertainty, frequently stronger than most other addictions. The strongest behavioral and belief addictions for many people appear in the religious area. This is due in part, to the deep personal meaning derived from examining profound social, spiritual and religious issues; as well as a bonding to a cultural and family religion. The issues of an after life and purpose of life transcend for many people the life they live on this planet. We note the increasing tendency to give up life for an after life, and fulfilling one's purpose in life by death; (Currently most notable in the conflict in Iraq and also expressed in past conflicts).

The sanctity of life is diminished, when we give up life for the after life, and find our purpose in life, in death.

One of the most important human attributes that serves to anchor people to a rigid outlook, making them closed minded and intolerant of difference, is an overriding emotional intensity, that overwhelms other sensibilities, including our inherent wisdom, an important guide for people. Emotional Intensity {abbreviation EI} is a much sought after quality in many cultures and certainly in our own. It is a necessary quality in competitive situations which demand winners and losers, such as athletic games and warfare events both national and domestic. EI serves to generate strong bonds and allegiance among people cementing an often unquestioning loyalty and camaraderie unifying and bonding members in a powerful way. In the current national and international political scenes, allegiance to political parties, tribal and ethnic groups, belief systems, and single issue political groups are the basis of support overriding the quality of the argument, or "information value" of the ideas. Energizing the political base is the recipe for success, and the successful leader is the one with the ability to elicit intense emotions often initiated with an inflammatory appeal. This type of an appeal raises the emotional intensity of the political base and effects individual members in a variety of ways. For example, recent understanding of a Biofeedback Loop as a biological mechanism highlights the interconnectedness of what used to be considered separate and discrete biological systems. The emotional system can effect the immune system which than returns an effect to the emotions. The feedback system is circular in nature. When people are continually bombarded with emotionally charged rhetoric, the same biofeedback system opporates to shape a psychobiological profile which seeks out and is influenced by the emotional intensity of arguments rather than the information value. Furthermore, prolonged emotional intensity will drain one's health and wellbeing. In the 21st century this is a recipe for disaster. Acceleration in weaponry, and the acceleration in emotional intensity are two of the most dangerous challenges facing humankind. We need to introduce an epiphamoneous feedback system based upon a higher consciousness, recognizing the interdependence of all people, to offset the more primitive consciousness of "winner take all" (and its my side that better win). With that goal in mind it is almost time to begin our journey, but not before we consider this final unifying idea which places an overall perspective upon most of the previous material.

Being a "winner" creates a "loser" unless you compete against your self.

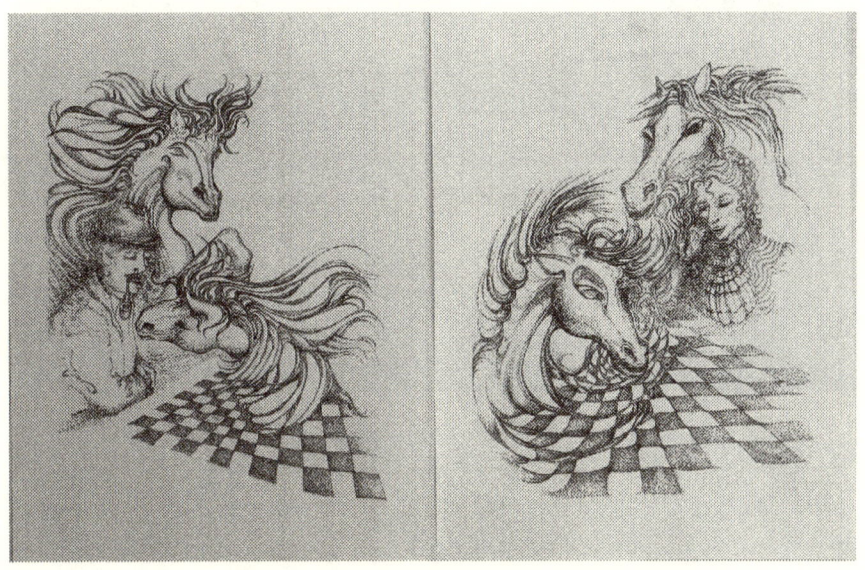

Appealing to emotions rather than understanding, is a recipe for disaster in the 21st century.

THE AGE OF
SYNCROHNICITY

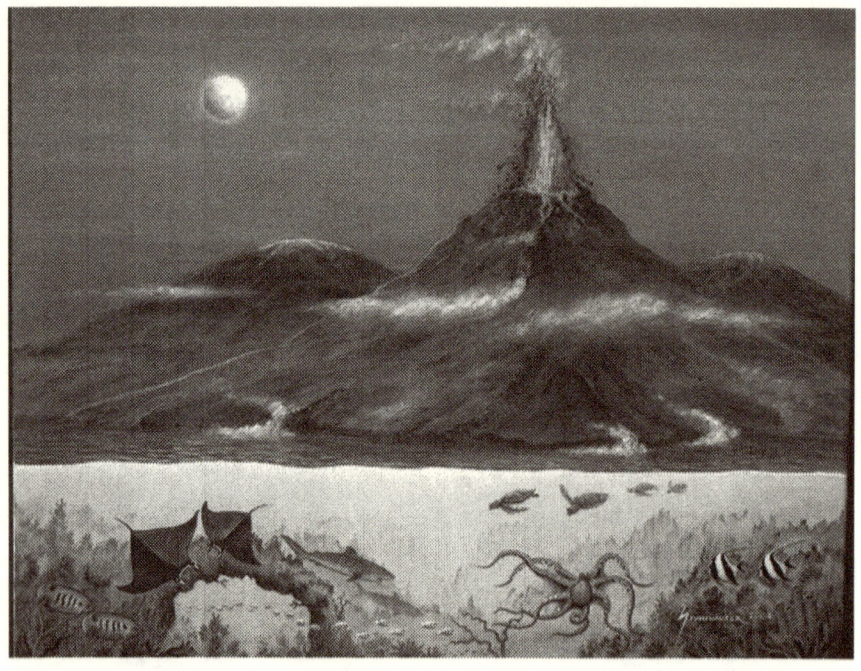

art by jerome stumphauzer

From a spiritual perspective, everything in the universe shares a common denominator, from inner and outer space, from macro to micro level, from animate to inanimate form, and for all planetary life, and evolutionary development.

In a previous section we noted a history of major conceptual shifts in human consciousness reflecting changes in the way we know, and how we explain our experience of life upon this planet. These were significant alterations in our mapping of the territory of human experience. We are now in the midst of such a shift. When these epistemological shifts occur there is always a mixture of the previous conceptual maps which continues to persists even to the present. (For example, one can still find elements of supernatural explanation as the underlying rationale of current events). New concepts help us to appreciate, understand, and experience our lives with greater and more sensitive awareness. The concept of synchronicity affords us this opportunity. Synchronicity relates to the field of energy which is generated by all life forms as well as inanimate objects which capture and reflects a connective energy that unifies and influences all. The energy exists in the air we breath, the land we live upon, the objects we possess, and the houses we inhabit. It is in our recounting of history, the clothes we wear and the food we eat. It is everywhere including our thoughts and emotions. The following examples illustrate this synchronicity principle. Recent experiments in Japan have shown that human emotions and thoughts influence the arrangements of water molecules in small containers of water. In the book Secret Life Of Plants the author describes the effects of human thought upon plant growth. Various accounts and publications have described animal behavior which has transcended time and space so that other animals suddenly exhibit the same behavior without opportunity to learn by contact. At a personal level; most of us have experienced the upsetting effects of a dramatic shift in the energy field after the 9/11 attack, and the cascade of consequences that followed. Counseling support was needed by many over a period of time to regain a measure of emotional balance to deal with an energy field contaminated by intense upsetting emotions. In a less intense manner, many of us can recount the effects of various places and physical surroundings upon our emotions, often at an intuitive level. We connect with, and join with our surroundings, feeling the the quality of energy inherent in the architecture of buildings and decor, as well as the natural elements of the great outdoors. Close prox-

imity creates rhythmic connections. Some examples of people and
things that harmonize rhythms when in close proximity include heart
cells in petri dishes beating at the same time and frequency; womens
menstrual cycles, when women live in close contact, and certain
machines in the close presence of other machines.

*What then is separation when we acknowledge an intimate connection to a
universal presence?*

These synchronicity fields vary in the quality of connective energy
that pervades various geographic areas and populations within those
areas, although energy fields are not limited to a given area. Much of
the intense entrenched turmoil and conflict within the Mideast can be
understood as resulting from centuries old tribal and religious warfare,
occupation, exploitation, torture, etc. that leaves a legacy of a hostile,
vindictive energy field that shapes and contaminates the inhabitants of
that region. This is often called the history of that region, or a cultural
narrative; after all, what is history, but a description in part of an
enduring regional synchronicity field with the resulting cultural details
(Of course that is not the whole story). All political, religious, cultural,
and ethnic groups generate, and are shaped by their shared connective
energy field which influences their behavior, attitudes, and world view.
The differences between these groups imbedded within different syncrohnicity fields are often an underlying source of conflict, often justi-
fied by a rationale designed to place each side in the "right".

We are all players on the Synchronicity Field.

A REFLECTING PAUSE

In the preparation phase of the journey we explored a number of historical, psychological, biological and social developments which have become ingrained in our cultures determining much of how we map our personal and social realities. The effects upon human kind have been mixed in that an explosion of scientific knowledge and technological development has yielded significant benefits to a large portion of humanity but certainly not to all. As we have entered an age of accelerating acceleration, the previous knowledge and attitude mind set is less able to guide us in dealing with the exploding complexity of the 21st century. Old rigid answers are not effective solutions to rapidly changing problems which increasingly impact our planet and its inhabitants. The challenges are formidable for there are many elements that keep us set in our views, attitudes, and behavior dealing with our internal and external life. At an early age, we all begin a journey of discovering and knowing. A cultural-family connection shapes our sense of who we are, and how we search, and that "shaping" needs to be understood from a mind-body-spirit perspective rather than a right-wrong, victim view. It is a complex picture never fully developed or understood; recall the adage of embarking upon a conscious journey of not knowing who you are. With that in mind let us take a pause that reflects.

Anything we focus upon, we magnify in our lives.

We began by examining the nature of explanation integrating the historical differences between two schools of Greek Philosophy, one concerned about "truth" the other concerned about the effects of the explanation upon the human condition. The concept of "Information Value" is an attempt to combine these positions being aware of both

41

perspectives so as to examine the source of the information as well as
the accuracy and lack of distortion, some of the qualities of truth. We
were reminded of two pitfalls in our journey, premature knowledge
and consciousness closure. Knowing the answer stops the search, and
limiting our search to a single method of inquiry and approach to
explanation shrinks the journey to a few steps. We are beginning to
appreciate some of the powerful forces that maintain our sense of who
and what we are, and how we seem to be controlled by those same
forces. We are connected to our culture, our family, our religion and
the various groups and mind shaping media that directly and indirectly
effect us. These forces effect us in a variety of ways by creating neurobi-
ological and psychobiological addictions that keep us fixed in our
beliefs, opinions, internal conversations, perceptions, body posture,
etc. We retain the same perceptual and psychological filters for viewing
reality as well as a rigid framing structure for relating the reality story to
our selves and others. Consequently rather than looking for valuable
information to <u>inform</u> (the root word of information), we look for
information <u>to confirm</u> our beliefs. (confirmation rather than information). This creates an expression of a psychobiological addiction to a
certain body chemistry resulting in strongly held views, beliefs and
similar repeating emotions. Additionally, much of our beliefs and
information are influenced by an either/or polarity which is the legacy
of an excluded middle definition of "truth". This tends to add a divisive and competitive flavor to much of our discussions serving to maintain distance, separation, and a rigid polarity about ideas. It's
important to note that humans are the only planetary life form that
will kill each other over words and ideas, and the language used frequently survives the original user. Language used in the present carries
over as a legacy for the future, and often creates an ongoing history of
social, political, and religious strife. It is the energy within the language
that has played an historical role in human affairs. Finally, we recognize an emergence into a new conceptual revolution or epistemological
shift into the age of Syncrohnicity which highlights a compelling con-

nection between our inner environment with our outer world. The impact of these various energy fields exert a most powerful impact upon human and planetary history. Some of these factors and forces that contribute to the quality of connective energy fields have been detailed in the above material, with the understanding that, nothing is the whole story in an emerging story.

Thoughts and ideas can leave an emotional legacy for future generations.

EMBARKING UPON THE EPIPHAMONIOUS JOURNEY

The journey of life depends upon where you travel, and how you are as a traveler.

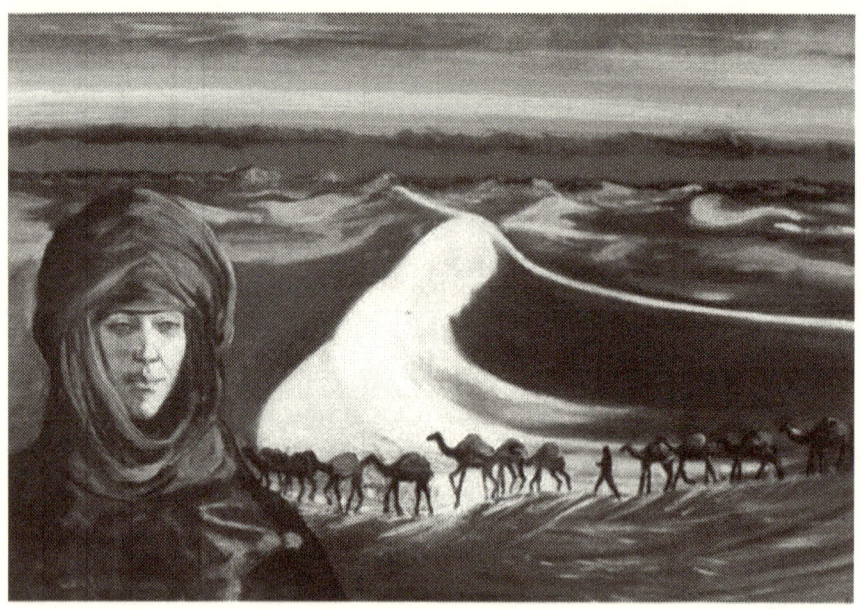

art by Scott Cumming

The nature of a journey is to explore unfamiliar landscapes, an adventure of discovery related to where you travel and how you are as a traveler. This journey deals with both aspects, to explore new ideas and ways to map your reality, and to increase your skills as a traveler. The two areas are intertwined; what you experience, depends upon who you are as well as where you travel.

We begin our journey by exploring a number of practices. A practice is defined as placing your attention, focus, and efforts upon a specific area so as to gain improvement and maximize benefit for the mind, body, and spirit. The nature of a practice suggests repeated efforts, along with an incubation period, allowing for time to develop increased proficiency. Among the requirements needed are patience, commitment and a gentle sense of loving purpose to ease the journey. (A sense of humor is also a big plus).

Practice takes practice.

A fundamental practice is the never ending process of raising awareness of the dynamic nature of who we are in an ever changing world. That practice requires further detailed explanation. There are many aspects to the concept of awareness. The word "awareness" is similar to the word "focus" in that both carry the idea of magnifying into consciousness. However focus carries the suggestion of a circumscribed area, a narrower set of goals, a more specific area of concentration. While there are many positive qualities to that concept, there is a significant downside; one can narrow their vision to a small part of the human affairs landscapes, missing the overall vista. Highlighting one aspect of any reality casts other elements into darkness; for example a relationship problem is often created when one partner fixates upon a particular goal becoming oblivious to other important concerns; or a single issue political groups losing sight of other important political issues. These are some of the dangers of a tunnel vision approach to life, being overly focused upon one's personal goals to the detriment of other important qualities of life. In contrast to the concept of focus, the idea of awareness is more inclusive, directed toward a more global, comprehensive and unified territory. It implies both a state of being—of who and what we are—and a process of becoming—one's evolutionary growth process. The "who" relates, in part, to the qualities we have as individuals, the mixture of compassion, love,sensitivity, greed, fearfulness, hostility, etc. In the physical world it comprises both our personal and social identities. The "what" relates to our basic nature. Are we human beings having a spiritual experience, or spiritual beings having a human experience. The former elevates the importance of the physical world, the latter emphasizes the intangible, metaphysical side. Which ever position is emphasized, will influence how we travel the highway of life. Our sense of "being" and "becoming" can also be considered as we think about our future transformation in relation to death, certainly one of the great mysteries of life, and perhaps another adventure of who we are and where we are going in our after life.

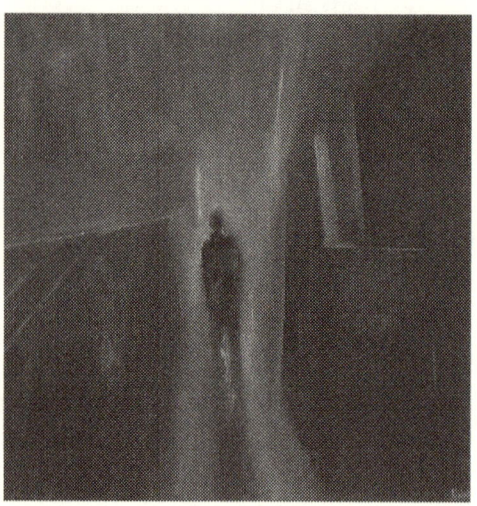

Art by Norman W Merrill

Being Love is not necessarily being in Love.

Another aspect of awareness relates to the "taking in" of information, experience,and energy at a mind-body-spirit level; which crosses the level from "unaware" into the levels of "dimly aware" (not able to put it into words), and "fully aware" (able to express it in a conscious fashion). It forms the underpinning of every other practice to follow. The practice is in the raising of awareness, increasing one's sensitivity, and expanding one's consciousness in areas health, wellbeing, spiritual growth, and enhancing the quality of planetary life.

One basic practice is in the broad area of communication which also carries with it the ideas of connection and feedback. In this practice arena we begin by awareness of "mind-body" or intrapersonal communication (within the person). The mind communicates with words, ideas, thoughts, and concepts. The body communicates with feelings, sensations, and other sensory responses. By heightening our awareness we focus upon how our thoughts and ideas effect our feelings, recognizing positive thoughts create positive feelings, neutral thoughts create neutral feelings and negative thoughts create negative feelings. We recognize the effects upon our bodies and our overall health created by the "energy of our thinking", as well as our often repeating internal dialog. Conversely, by examining body communication we gather, information about our life style and living habits ranging from our <u>nutritional,</u> (life supporting quality or lack there of, of the foods we eat,) <u>social</u> (supportive, energy draining, or toxic associations) and <u>physical</u> (amount and quality of exercise and movement we include in our daily lives.) It is the recognition and increasing attention given to this feedback situation of mind/body talk that forms a basic practice, remembering that anything we focus upon we magnify in our lives. With this increasing sensitivity we can expect improved health and well being, and a heightening of our intuition and creativity.

The mind talks with words and ideas, the body talks with feelings and sensations. Together they form an important conversation to be understood.

The above saying is an important principle that underlies any journey of transformation and needs to be fully explored both as a tool for change and spiritual growth; as well as a basic understanding of human behavior and consciousness. The combination of mind/body communication is the basic component of our emotions. An emotion is a pairing of a physical sensation with a thought or concept, For example, as a result of an event or experience one responds with a variety of physical sensations as a physical response to that event. One than labels those physical sensations and feelings with a mental word or concept to make it comprehensible and understandable. We than use labels like fear, anger, love, boredom, etc.; most of which are the names for emotions and the basis for our emotional reactions (acting out of anger love or fear or any emotional mix). Much of our behavior has an underlying emotional basis frequently unknown or unclear to us. Often we disguise our basic emotional feelings with an explanation that is acceptable to our selves and others. The basic practice is to increase our awareness of our emotional motivations and than to choose from a more spiritual mix, based upon love, compassion, service, support, etc. We support the moral evolution of ourselves and others, recognizing our basic connection to each other.

The internal dialog is another area of intrapersonal communication; that ongoing inner conversation that can be such a bother as we ruminate over past grievances and future fears. The level, frequency, and intensity, is a measure of personal stress. It is like an emotional fever, the greater the frequency and intensity, the greater the emotional discomfort. There are ways to lessen this infernal internal dialog including a variety of meditation practices which help in quieting the mind. These practices are worthwhile, readily available and will be briefly discussed in a later section. As part of this practice we will explore a mental process to lower the level of internal preoccupation. The practice is creating an increasing detachment to the dialog. A repeating internal dialog is like a circular freeway with very few exits, going round and round continuously repeating the same ideas. It gets you nowhere except tired and stressed. A way of leaving this freeway is by naming the freeway using a label that in some way describes this well traveled road. Every time you re enter think of the name rather than driving forth on the freeway. For example being stuck in a circle of past anger or grievance is similar to a court room drama with a judge, jury, and opposing attorneys were one is defending one's self and attacking another. This is a very common internal dialog. You might label this as "courtroom", or "red light" or any other creative name to prevent yourself from entering, or being able to quickly exit once entered. Using a label or name is a way of detaching and creating space from that disturbing reoccurring thinking. Upsetting and disturbing thoughts also effect the body as part of a mind/body connection.

Negative emotions anchor painful memories

Most, if not all upsetting internal dialogs are emotionally based. and often are the result of painful memories. <u>Emotions are the basic glue to anchor upsetting memories and thoughts to our consciousness.</u> Painful memories relate to past experiences and often carry the basic emotion of anger and its many variations (resentment, hate, guilt or self anger, etc.). Painful thoughts of the future while not memories often carry fear based emotions such as fear, anxiety, apprehension, etc. Often we are advised to forget about upsetting memories but since they are embedded into our consciousness, they persist over time. It is in the lessening and defusing of the emotions that will lessen the upsetting nature of the memory. There is a technique to do this. Rather than focus upon the remembered event, explore your emotions and feelings related to the memory. Maintaining your focus upon your feelings instead of the details of the event, will lessen the upset even though the memory remains. Relaxing the physical sensations will lessen the bond of painful feelings to cognitive thoughts and memories.

An additional remedy to lessen the impact of repetitive thoughts is to internally repeat the phrase; "out of mind and body" when ever these unwanted thought arise. This will lessen the impact of these thoughts upon mind/body wellbeing. Unless there is an environmental trigger for these thoughts, their upsetting nature will eventually dissipate. Because of the mind/body unity, one can also utilize physical techniques ranging from various physical exercises as well as specific exercises related to eye movement to lessen and extinguish the pain associated with memories and thoughts. The eye movement technique typically requires the guidance of a trained psychotherapist.

Another basic intrapersonal communication practice is a powerful source of personal guidance. That is a practice of discovery of the inner wisdom, sometimes experienced as an intuitive feeling or inner voice, which is part of our spiritual inheritance. There is a saying "knowledge is learned, wisdom is discovered". One need not go to a college to learn wisdom. On the contrary, solitude, reflection, and quiet periods away from the distractions of much of our lives, creates the arena for this very important practice. Our environment can be an important force in supporting or detracting from this practice, providing both the stimulation and the personal space to nourish our progress.

Spiritual evolution is not about redoing the past but changing the present.

1. As we relate to people, interpersonal communication occurs between people at many different levels and layers at the same moment. There are at least five levels or layers worthy of attention within this practice; four of which can be illustrated in the form as a "communication box". The fifth level will be discussed separately but nevertheless is an important component of all face to face communication and contact. Verbal communication can be examined from the actual words that are used, (verbal) as well as the body language of movement and expression (nonverbal). Each communication level carries significant meaning and often it is the nonverbal that creates the most impact. In other words, it is not only what we say, but how we say it. When we speak, we most often believe we speak with a specific intention, but frequently there are unintentional elements that are communicated as well. Verbal communication can not only communicate information but

express our emotional state. These are four levels of communication; verbal, nonverbal, intended, unintended. At a fifth level, communication is a form of "energy transmission" which can have significant effects upon the health and wellbeing of both communicating parties; and can have enduring effects beyond a simple two person exchange. This will be discussed further, but now we will examine one of many ways people talk in the following table.

COMMUNICATION BOX

	Verbal	Non Verbal
Intended	Purposeful communication, such as questions answers, specific requests, giving directions, etc. These are fully conscious responses.	Fully conscious physical responses such as gestures,conscious facial expressions, eye movement, striking of a pose, etc.
Non Intended	Excessive repeating of certain words or instructions; dwelling upon certain topics or ideas. Slips of the tongue; stumbling over certain words or phrases, etc.	Unintentional communication of emotion, mood, energy level by body posture, eye movement, throat tension, tightness in body, nervous gestures, etc.

You cannot __not__ communicate, for that is a communication.[1]

The practice is to increase awareness at all of the above areas including unintended communication, recognizing the power of the words you use, and the short and long term effects your words have upon others. There is a saying that one can not, not communicate; that non communication is a communication. There is much communication that surrounds unintended verbal and nonverbal exchanges some of which is described in the unintended level of the above box. There are many other ways of verbal and nonverbal behavior exert profound

---

1.   An apt saying from the Palo Alto Group; D. Jackson, G. Bateson, P. Watzla-wock, et.al.

effects upon people including the following fifth level of communication which relates to the transmission of energy. We are all sensitive to varying degrees to the state of a persons energy, whether its high, medium, or low, agitated, or calm, strong or weak, etc. Many healers are able to sense the energy within and surrounding a person. Kirlian photography is a method of photographing the energy fields that flow as well as surround us. People are effected by these energy fields both in a positive and or a negative way often without being aware of their impact. As our sensitivity and awareness increases in this area, new opportunities for healing are presented for both our selves and others, as energy can often be controlled. Energy flow and its transmission is another vital area for study in that all living organisms exist within energy fields; including the earth as a life sustaining planet.

In communication, the tip of the iceberg are the words we use. What lies beneath holds the deeper meaning.

The reader is reminded that information often has a static quality or feeling, in part because the reader some what passively absorbs the ideas hopefully with some reflection. After the process of reflection and acceptance, begins a process of incorporating the ideas into one's behavior, which is the key component in any practice. It is the action taken, that forms a key element in the practice, along with non judgmental awareness. This next practice speaks to this purpose. We all have a variety of responses to the ebb and flow of daily events. When events are upsetting and painful, we call upon our "coping mechanisms" to deal with the situation, and maintain our emotional balance. Life offers many large and small events which can upset that balance, such as feeling uncertain and anxious over the most seemingly innocuous situations. It is the confidence we feel in our own abilities to deal with situations that provides the most comfort. We can enhance our overall social effectiveness and personal balance by increasing our Repertoire of Responses which includes the range, the variety, and the quality of our responses to any given life situation. The practice is remaining sufficiently detached so as to observe yourself and the situation, to remain flexible, to avoid making right/wrong judgments or engage in a competitive contest. You have the greatest control over your own behavior. You cannot force others to freely behave in the way you desire, but you can influence them by your actions. By acting out of a sense of Love, and a concern for the best interests of all, you will increase the positive quality of your responses. Maintaining a proper motivation of healing, improving, and serving all concerned, is a key. Opening one's self to new responses with motivation combining the force of the mind and spirit is one of the most effective way of expanding your Repertoire of Responses.

Acting out of a sense of love and concern for all, increases the positive quality of your response

No one says we have to walk on this journey. The 21st century offers some benefits as well as challenges; we can drive! As we journey forth in our car we notice the sudden appearance of a red warning light on our dash board. Do we take a hammer, smash out the light and keep driving? Or do we pull over, stop the car and try to figure out what's wrong? The warning light is a communication that all is not well with the car. We usually do not continue on our journey without making corrections. Yet in our own lives that is frequently what we do. We ignore our pain and discomfort and most often try to block out painful feelings, taking a pill to eliminate our discomfort or self-medicating with drugs or alcohol.

Symptoms are an invaluable communication about our lifestyle: our physical, psychological, spiritual, social, and nutritional lifestyle. When we respond to the communication by making appropriate life style changes, the symptoms having served their purpose will lessen and eventually disappear. This is the basic underlying principle and practice of a holistic health approach, lifestyle change rather than solely controlling symptoms without learning from our pain.

Pain is the fuel for change. People who don't get good mileage need more.

Given this understanding, the burden of maintaining and improving our health shifts from a paid outsider to the individual. We can hire a consultant or teacher to provide necessary resources, information and expertise but the basic control and responsibility remains with the individual or "patient". This is not to say that we do not seek pain control or ignore intractable pain. Medical advice and help can be invaluable for pain control and symptom management. Rather we broaden our understanding of the purpose and function of pain; first to get our attention and second to bring about change. Pain is the fuel for change. Some people get good mileage from their pain making change less painful; while others less "pain-fuel efficient" require more. We strive to require less pain-fuel and become more "fuel-less", If we ignore the fundamental communication and purpose of pain the symptoms become "loud and more intrusive". If we continue to ignore,we risk becoming "prematurely recycled".

The true source of healing lies within each individual.

This "holistic practice" emphasizes the true source of healing is within each individual rather than something outside of oneself. Supplements and medicine can be very necessary supports to improve and maintain health, but they are not the full story for health and wellness. Combining a healthy lifestyle with prudent supplementation of vitamins, minerals, herbs, and other natural products, and any necessary prescribed medication is an intelligent approach to good health and wellness.

Health and wellness are not limited to a pill box approach.

As a population, we are increasingly being "educated" by a mass media that is driven by profit which in turn can subtly influence our attitudes toward health. For example, the various antacid ads showing a person in gastric distress after eating a variety of "garbage foods", rather than improving our diet (no profit to the sponsor) the answer is to buy the sponsor's product so that we can "garbage up" without discomfort. As enlightened and responsible consumers of information, we must combine the knowledge of science with the wisdom of our own body and spirit. Heeding our own body's feelings and reactions, as well increasing our own intuitive awareness, are the truer guides to health and wellbeing. The practice is learning from our pain, understanding the underlying communication, and being fuel efficient in the use of pain for lifestyle change. Included in that practice is increasing our own ability to respond (responsibility) and assume greater control and direction over our health and wellbeing. We must also increase our awareness of how our personal struggles relate to the larger global issues that effect us all. We are like individual waves in a larger ocean, each wave is unique with its own particular qualities and direction that finally ends on a distant shore, yet all are part of the same ocean. We must increasingly extend a nurturing concern to our environment which is intimately connected to all of us both metaphorically and physically. Finally, we begin to initiate personal and planetary changes based upon qualities of love, compassion, spiritual understanding, and a sense of humor (for comfort and balance.)

There is an adage in Naturopathic medicine, diseases of the mind, go through the body, diseases of the body go through the mind. This next practice eliminates the separation of body and mind. This is a practice of conscious movement. Usually, when one thinks of conscious movement one thinks of movement with a purpose frequently to accomplish some specific task or increasing one's skill in a sport. In this practice the emphasis. Is upon the effects of the movement upon the body/mind. It is the difference between playing playing a game of tennis where movement is designed to hit the ball over a net in a manner to defeat the opponent; contrasted to practicing yoga where one is focused upon the feelings and effects of the movement upon the body, mind,mood and energy. The nature of this movement practice is to

feel and explore these effects. One adopts a different mindset, consequently the results are different. It is similar to assuming a yogic mentality to the movement, which is decidedly not competitive or
purposive other than exploring the mind-body effects. With this basic
mentality as our guide we can now explore a variety of movement
which comprise this next practice.

Diseases of the mind, attend to the body. Diseases of the body attend to the
mind.

Movement can be examined from many different aspects, each magnify certain qualities and gains but nothing is a total package. There is
a certain level of creativity and experimentation that can be employed
in this practice which differs from a set training approach. Both
approaches can be used, each creating different kinds of movements,
qualities and benefits for your mind/body. The cardinal rule is "LIS-
TEN TO YOUR BODY" as you engage in all movements.

Movement can exercise the mind, body, and spirit at the same time.

Movement and exercise can be located on a continuum ranging
from targeting the physical body to targeting the intuitive and metaphysical side, with a mixture of benefits at the midpoint. Targeting the
physical body would include primarily weight training exercises
including the use of weights, exercise machines, pull ups, core muscle
training and other exercises that target particular muscle groups. The
primary purpose is for strength training, muscle development and
body shaping, frequently for competitive purposes. The benefits
Include increased muscle strength as well as some emotional calming
benefits resulting from strenuous physical activity. The arena for much
of this exercise format is typically a gym, sports club or other training
area. Examples of mixed exercises benefiting body/mind are: jogging
swimming, and other long distance repetitive exercises. Benefits
include cardiovascular enhancement, strength and endurance building,
as well as psychological benefits such as a quieting the mind, experienc-

ing a "runners high" or a slight sense of euphoria, and generally experiencing an overall feeling of tranquility. Near the metaphysical/intuitive side, we have a variety of exercises and movements that offer a range of life enhancing responses, Practices like Tai Chi, Chi Gung, various forms of yoga, Sufi dancing and chanting etc. provide some physical gains as well as a range of intuitive and metaphysical benefits, Some of these include emotional stabilization, altered states of consciousness, epiphamonious experiences or moments of clarity, and heightened physical and emotional energy states. Physical benefits include increased body flexibility, range of motion, enhanced balance, and cardiac and pulmonary gain. These forms are often practiced with like minded people in a supportive physical environment.

All of the above physical practices are in an environment generally designed for a particular movement regime, often under the direction of a trainer, teacher, or facilitator. A creative adventure is in the developing and integrating an "exercise experience" into your every day routine. One can exercise while in the shower, brushing ones teeth, walking, standing, exercising in front of a mirror, etc. all of which can cover a full spectrum of body-mind benefit. The techniques include muscle tensing, isometric and breath exercises, laughing exercise, stretching, balancing, toning (use of sounds to create vibrations in certain parts of one's body) and facial exercises which should be a component to all of the above exercises. Laughing and the use of sounds are ways to work on the inner body including vital inner organs and glands. Recall that facial exercises will balance one's emotional state and mood. Its the taking of vitamin S, the silly pill which lessens depression, lowers stress, and in general rebalanced one's emotional portfolio. Facial exercise will also tone facial skin thereby creating an inexpensive facial treatment to retard wrinkles and aging lines.

If the head is corrupt the body will follow.

What is needed to facilitate this creative practice is an epiphamonious tool kit. Some of the tools you already posses (at a bargain price) others can be purchased at a modest cost. A very easy to use tool is laughing which is a simple exercise that must be approached as an exercise. You simply start laughing (preferably alone, or if in India a laughing group) No outside funny stimulus is needed. One concentrates on the effects of laughing upon the body, feeling the sensations and tensions created by an altered state of breathing and muscle movement This exercise alone has shown benefit to strengthen the immune system, perhaps by "working" the thymus gland which is essential to that system, Body locks, (not to be confused with smoked salmon) is a centuries old practice of squeezing or tightening specific muscles or muscle groups for a short time, relaxing and repeating. Let your body guide you as to tempo. Many women are familiar with this practice when they do the Kagel exercises to strengthen their pelvic floor. Men recognize the same benefits for their prostate. These locks can be used throughout the body to strengthen various muscles, and are part of certain yoga practices to contain energy. Slow movement while tensing related muscles is another highly effective way to build muscles strength without any aids.

Perhaps the most versatile tool in our tool box is the inflatable exercise ball with an appearance similar to a beach ball. They come in different sizes. Most stores try to fit you to a "right size". This author's experience is that different sizes offer somewhat different exercise experience, and more than one ball can be used at the same time to create a variety of exercises. The ball can be used as a punching bag, kicking bag, squeezing bag, rapid hitting bag, bouncing bag (some writers believes that the particular bouncing exercise may have benefits at the cellular level). One can roll upon a ball to increase flexibility and balance, a ball to control one's effort when doing push ups, and a ball to aid in achieving certain yoga positions and meditative states, just to name a few benefits. Perhaps one of the most effective is exercising the "core muscle group" consisting of lower back,thighs, abdomen, hips, and related muscle groups, which are important for stability balance, and overall strength. In addition,the balls are excellent for strengthening, toning, and increasing range of motion for the neck. Certainly one of the most effective and versatile exercise implements and inexpensive as well.

This next exercise tool is the resistance cord, and resistance band, both serve the same purpose, however the band is more compact but generally less durable, and somewhat more limited in its use. One typically is not able to stand on the band which limits lower body exercise, The particular advantage to these tools are their portability. They are easily carried with hands free, and you can walk or hike and have the ability to use your private gym outdoors. It's great! The resistance cord can also be used in conjunction with other exercise machines for a more total workout. It is vitally important to be cleared by an appropriate health professional before undertaking any significant exercise program,including any of the above.

As mentioned earlier the muscles of the face are strongly connected to our emotions and mood. The following exercise is a way to improve one's mood, and no prescription is needed. One needs to be alone and be sure that your voice does not carry to others unless they are informed. Open your mouth wide by dropping your jaw and making the sound yaaaa; repeat as needed, Next, purse your lips,saying the sound woowoowoowoo; repeat as needed. Finally, contort your face into a wide silly grin repeating the word yi yi yi yi etc. Repeat as necessary. Focus on the feeling of feeling silly, and expand it, Now give your self a hug and kiss your arm or shoulder......you silly person.

Do not squander an opportunity to be silly.

I leave the reader with this final movement practice which I consider to be very vital but which is given insufficient attention in most gyms, and practice regimens. It is the purposeful and conscious use of breath; a subtle connection to our forebears, since we breath the same atmospheric components as they did in their lives which may in fact convey their energy to the present. It is known that the breath conveys emotional energy; and certain cultures in the past have made it a practice to smell the breath of their guests. Our language captures this idea when we mention the idea of a breath that smells of fear. Biblical stories relate mystical stories of the use of breath to give life. It is largely an unexplored area although currently there are various breathing techniques that are taught and used today. Only one technique will be explored in some detail as an example of the power of breath. There is a story which accompanies this particular practice which is worth telling because it illustrates at least two principles; one of learning; the other the nature of this practice. Recently, I met a physician who was a speaker at a Holistic Health conference who related a personal experience that changed his life and medical practice in a most dramatic and profound fashion. He was a cardiologist with a very successful and lucrative practice when he contracted a life threatening disease. He followed the usual course of medical treatment without any significant benefit, left his practice, and finally went to Mexico with his wife to spend his last days finding what ever little satisfaction he could in his dying body. His wife left to return to the the States for a short period, and while alone and in a weaken condition, he managed a short walk into the neighborhood. He met a person who he described as a "Yogi" who during their conversation labeled him a "stupid doctor" after the doctor had related the details of his current terminal condition. After recovering from the affront and professional ego shock of being called a "stupid doctor" the Yogi introduced him to a series of rapid breathing exercises which over an extended period of time led to his recovery and consequently a dramatic change, enabling him to return to his medical setting and practice. He then showed me a particular breathing exercise, which we both did. I recognized the exercise as "The Breath Of Fire" which is a fundamental practice in Kundalini Yoga, a form that I had practiced for a limited period many years past. He reacquainted me with a past experience providing a new appreciation and an increased awareness for this form of yoga. This is a principle of "Spiral Learning" wherein one returns to a past experience and derives a deeper and more sensitive appreciation and understanding of that experience, similar to the image of a spiral moving deeper in essentially in the same area. Reoccurring experiences offer an opportunity for a greater understanding and are not to be seen as a waste of time and dismissed with a curt "I already knew that". Often when one does not learn from a reoccurring experience one is assuming the role of a "victim" a common outcome from failing to learn from repetitive behavior.

The quality of breath reflects and effects one's mind/body state.

The actual practice is the esoteric use of the breath. I use the word "esoteric" which conveys the meaning of "being understood by a select few" often for a spiritual purpose. Historically there have been various breathing practices and exercises contained within various specialized groups which were generally not shared with the larger community. These practices were often limited to the members of religious and spiritual sects. Currently, these ideas are being spread, but generally remain largely unknown unless you are in a particular sport, martial arts, or yogic practice. Within these practices, conscious breathing is used for specific results such as to increase strength, relaxation, body flexibility, focus, and balance. Attention is given to the nature of the breath, whether shallow or deep, breath on the inhalation or exhalation, rapid or slow, breath held or slowly released; these are some of the conscious variations of breath control. The Breath Of Fire as practiced in Kundalini Yoga is a powerful technique which builds and extends a powerful energy through out the mind/body which can release an energy that lies dormant in the body. Years ago, a patient was referred to me from a mental health center that was baffled by his "psychiatric illness" He was a workman on the Alaska pipe line which was designed to carry oil to the States. Because of the solitude and the isolation of his work, he began a constant practice of the Breath Of Fire to occupy his time while on the job. In Kundalini terms he "uncurled the serpent" which released this dormant energy which lies within us all. He was unprepared to deal with that energy, which led to his return to California as a"mental patient". Fortunately, with direction he recovered to return to his work. One has to be oriented to the use of this breathing technique although the technique is simple enough. It consists of a series or rapid breaths inhaled through the nose and exhaled through the nose. Extensive use can lead to unexpected results as in the above story. However, in the case of the physician who recovered from his illness, careful use of this breathing technique can be helpful. It may also provide cardiovascular benefit to people with impaired mobility, and limited ability to exercise, with approval from your medical practitioner.

Like any other mother, the earth provides food to nourish her offspring, and we need to be in harmony with those offerings.

This next practice illustrates the profound connection we have to our planet and unfortunately it has been unrecognized, or ignored by most people. It has to do with food, and no, it's not about dieting. The initial idea was first put forth by the ancient Chinese as part of a Taoist philosophy related to the nature of food. Food combines energy from four sources and carries that energy to the consumer. (excuse the modern language) Food carries energy from the earth (soil), water, air, and sun. If any of those sources are deficient or contaminated, the energy of the food is adversely effected. Poor soil, contaminated air or water, insufficient sun; any combination lowers the energy (read nutritional) value of the food. Food preparation and processing can further diminish nutritional value. As a Taoist monk might say, "In order to be in nourishing harmony with planetary offerings of food, we should keep to the natural state of affairs." In other words raw, live and unprocessed or limited processed food are likely to carry the most necessary energy for life. The Taoist tradition also describes the nature of the energy carried by different foods, and no its not the four food groups or food pyramid. Food that fall from the sky such as many types of fruits carry a sedating or quieting energy; food that grows in the ground is balancing; and finally, food that travels along or close to the surface is energizing. People generally need a mix of foods but that mix should reflect one's stage in life as well as the nature and activity level of work. Its no accident that the US military generally serves three meat meals daily to support the intense physical energy level of military personnel, thereby using the energizing quality of food. From a health food perspective, it is important to recognize that preparation and processing can further diminish nutritional value.

In order to be in nourishing harmony with planetary offerings, we should keep to the natural state of affairs.

As an example of the effects of this subtle food energy upon people, this author had an experience of a new patient, a beginning graduate student who had been a vegetarian for many years complaining that she lacked the energy and the drive to survive graduate school. I recommended a dietary change to include meat to help provide a more aggressive energetic focus toward her studies. She later reported an increase in her energy and ability to focus on her studies. The principle is, the mix of food, which will support the direction in your life, for a given purpose and stage of life. For a contemplative and reflective direction consume less or no animal products; conversely for a high energy, physical focus, more animal products, although many vegetarians do report having sufficient energy. The reader is reminded that this is not the whole story, and there are many exceptions to these last statements, It is important to note that there are no right diets for all people at all times. The practice is for each traveler to discover the diet that will support there ever changing journey. One final note, The Taoist tradition does not consider a form of food energy that is an important factor in modern life, and that is the energy resulting from the motivations of the food growers and processesors. Food grown and processed purely for profit, will have a "pure profit energy" added to the food which will effect diet, nutritional health, and overall wellbeing of consumers. Taste can be manipulated and shaped to create food habits and addictions, a "Being Stuck" situation with food which nourishes the pure profit motive of the producer but which provides little or even adverse effects to the consumer, Raising one's awareness as to the motives of food producers and the resulting impact upon food energy or nutrition, is an important practice in creating a well fortified journey. Food and nourishment confirm a profound connection to our planet and to the universe in general. Even though we might find the universe overwhelming and foreign, we belong in that universe by being a family member of our planet. It can be a profound and comforting recognition for a never ending journey because where ever we travel we are ultimately still at home in our personal "center of the universe." As a family planetary member, we have a responsibility to all family members as well as to mother earth. At the very least, we should consider establishing elder abuse laws to protect our planet. If we fail, we will face disastrous natural consequences in the life sustaining qualities of our planet. <u>Planetary abuse translates to life abuse,</u> which implies a deeper and broader meaning to a "pro life" position.

Mother earth should be protected by elder abuse laws.

This last practice is perhaps one of the most vital, offering the potential for the most far reaching benefits for all. It relates to what often people think of as their "purpose in life" when one considers their future, and reason for existence. When one reflects upon their past, the idea of purpose changes to the idea of a "legacy left". Both views are important representing different stages of life as a platform for reflection. Which ever developmental stage that one pauses for reflection, it must include one's contribution to the synchronicity energy field. This includes the complex energy embedded in the cultural narrative or historical description and explanation of a given people or area. It is the pervasive emotional, spiritual, and psychic energy that is carried in words as well as the nature of expression which composes a significant proportion of the energy field. The practice is to continually increase your awareness of your contribution to the energy field as reflected by your actions, statements, emotional expressions, and your intentions. It is recognizing your unique and indelible contribution to an enduring field of energy that stays beyond your physical presence on earth.

What legacy will we leave for planetary life?

In order for an evolutionary change to occur in human consciousness a certain critical mass must occur so that sufficient numbers of people can, through their energy, create a shift in the all pervading synchronicity energy field supporting an evolutionary advance in human understanding and consciousness. An example of such a shift is described in the book The 100th Monkey which describes a sudden and major shift in animal behavior. Several small islands off the coast of Japan are inhabited by colonies of monkeys feeding primarily on the fruit from a particular tree. Fruit that had fallen from the tree was directly eaten until an older female monkey began washing the fruit in a nearby stream prior to eating. Other monkeys began copying her behavior until the entire group followed her behavior. The monkeys living on the adjacent islands almost spontaneously began exhibiting the same behavior even though there was no contact with monkeys from the initiating island. It seemed as if there was an all encompassing burst of new behavior in that population through some connecting communication field which altered monkey behavior. Borrowing a term from nuclear physics a "critical mass" had been reached which led to an "explosion" of changed behavior effecting the entire group. This type of shift is very different from the mass persuasion techniques used to manipulate people for personal interest by changing people's opinions and beliefs. This is often used by politicians, political leaders, marketing people, and the myriad of other persuaders pervading social and political change with a personal agenda. That approach often pollutes the synchronicity field with the self serving personal profiteering motivation which is carried by their attempts to persuade. There is an absence of morality in self serving persuasion. When one supports the integrity and ability of others to embark upon their own epiphamonious journey, in harmony with the interconnectedness of the whole, that is moral behavior. This last practice is to behave, act, and think, in an epiphamonious fashion in order to add your energy in support of the critical mass raising the level of human consciousness to the next evolutionary stage. It is a legacy of loving service to the all important energy field that connects us all.

There are not just laws embedded in the universe waiting to be discovered; there are agreements waiting to be made.

DESTINATION

We are embedded in an evolutionary process connected to a loving universe by a set of ever changing agreements.

1. There are not just laws embedded in the universe waiting to be discovered; there are agreements waiting to be made. The idea of a universal law related to the conception of the universe as a universal machine separate from the observer, is a mechanistic approach implying a likelihood of being controlled by man, once the mechanics are understood. The early scientists believed they could only use the tools of careful observation and measurement as a means to discover the immutable workings of the universe. This created a view of an uncompromising, controlling order for the inner and outer workings of the universe which governed man but could also be subject to control. It was an 18th century model which has survived into this time. The laws reflect the metaphor of an 18th century mechanical machine. What is currently needed is a betterphor expanding the limits of the previous metaphor,and the better metaphor is the idea of Universal Agreements. These are agreements waiting to be made with different travelers depending upon their spiritual and psychobiological stage as well as the level of technology that reflects their evolutionary development. The majority of people are governed by a system of beliefs which are based upon their psychological and social history. In that sense, beliefs carry a sense of "unchanging truth" based upon past experiences; devoid of the power for an individual to change the inevitable. They can convey a sense of powerlessness, helplessness, and hopelessness in ones ability to make significant life changes, if

strongly held. Beliefs foster a sense of acceptance of life with the idea of, "that's the way the world works". One can become imprisoned by a rigid belief system which stymies personal growth and evolutionary progress. Changing the idea of "beliefs" to "agreements" sets the stage for and evolutionary leap of consciousness wherein one creates a sense of empowerment to influence and foster an evolutionary journey. Every journey has a destination and this journey is no exception, and like everything else it is "<u>evolving</u>"(moving in a loving direction). We live within a set of agreements with an ever changing, evolving universe, and since we are profoundly connected in ways which we dimly understand, we are part of that evolutionary process. Simply stated, we are embedded in an evolutionary process connected to a loving universe by a set of ever changing agreements. The universe offers agreements which includes opportunities to change agreements. Since everything is connected, changing agreements changes the traveler as well. The agreements offered in part reflect our developmental level both in our state of consciousness and our state of technology which after all, is an extension of our consciousness. As humans, we evolve in a number of ways. We travel through various life stages from a dependent infant/child to an <u>interdependent</u> adult. Note that the concept of an <u>independent</u> adult is not used, since its similar to the idea of a single cell disconnected and isolated from adjoining cells, violating the idea of universal connection. At each developmental stage we live with agreements with the universe that reflect our stage of developing consciousness and ability. As our understanding evolves and our abilities grow, opportunities are offered to evolve those agreements in order to maintain an evolutionary balance with a universe that promotes loving growth. In a sense, the closer we come to realizing an agreement which fosters our own spiritual and evolutionary growth, the closer we come to a state of love. Conversely, the further we stray from universal agreements, the greater the discomfort and pain level, similar to discovering the qualities of a disappointed lover who seeks to encourage us into personal growth and more responsible behavior.

The closer we come to realizing an agreement with the universe the closer we come to a state of love. Conversely, the further we stray the greater the pain.

The question arises as to what kind of agreements have we made with the universe. This is the basic epistemological question relating to how we live our life and how we explain our life to ourselves and others. It is the basis of our beliefs, our sense of identity, an explanation of the past, and our sense of the future. It is our belief as to the nature of the universe, and our place within that universe, and to life in general. Whether we are unaware, dimly aware, or very aware, we act and think within those agreements. Which universe have we made our agreements with? Is it a "Deductive Universe" where we rely upon certain principles that have been given to us by "experts" in science and religion to explain the nature of worldly events and our role and responsibilities within that world. Is it a mechanical universe, where all the laws governing that great machine will be discovered by man and his increasingly accurate technology; with the promise of greater control over the uncertainties of nature that effect human and other life forms. Is it and "Energy Universe" whereby we and everything else are connected in often unknown ways. Is it a "Mysterious Universe" where everything is evolving including our understanding as to the basic nature of all; or is it a combination of the above ideas as well as some yet to be expressed? Each one of these views suggest a life stance, a way of existence, living one"s life in a certain fashion. It can be a life of obedience following the principles given to us by others. It can be a life of expectation that we as a life form will exert greater control of our destiny through our developing technology to solve our problems sometime in the future, so why worry now. Our definition of the universe includes a definition of our selves in terms of who we think we are, as well as how we live our lives. When we are in a loving relationship, we embark upon a journey of exploring who we are within the unfolding of that relationship. The elements of nurturing, love and pleasure form a binding and bonding connection. It can be orgasmic in nature as we are always pulled into the adventure of the present.

When you consciously choose the Universe to be your partner in an orgasmic relationship, you are committing yourself and your concern for the earth and all its family members, to an action of love, pleasure, and survival.

As with all lovers, the familiarity with an orgasmic sexual experience is common to all planetary life forms, otherwise they would not exist. There are at least two aspects to be considered in a sexual encounter. One is the drive for the physical pleasure of the experience and the other is to insure the survival of the species. Granted, there are many other purposes and elements to sexual encounters, but for the purpose of this discourse, the focus is upon personal pleasure and survival. A quality of a sexual orgasm is the riveting experience, drawing the participants into a highly focused concentrated awareness of an ecstatic moment. There is an ecstasy zone which is of short duration and intense of sensation. If a person is distracted, or thinking about some past or future issue, that orgasmic zone is evaded. Thinking about doing your laundry clothes you off to the zone. "Too much in the mind closes you off to the body", often the problem for an inorgasmic individual. There are other kinds and qualities of orgasmic experiences both of a sexual and nonsexual nature as well as a combination of both. One can be riveted to a piece of music or work of art which may elicit a variety of pleasure responses, as well as a moving emotional moment. In that experience, the time period is longer, and the person can respond without negating that orgasmic zone. The idea of an orgasmic experience and connection is not a single kind of experience but offers many variations and qualities certainly worthy of exploration. When you consciously choose The Universe to be your partner in establishing an orgasmic relationship, you are committing yourself, as well as your concern for the earth and all its family members, to an action of love, pleasure, and survival. Since we are a part of the universe, the search for orgasmic connection and universal agreement is within our selves That is the direction of our journey. As we evolve in our wisdom and understanding, we become capable of acting in a more <u>powerful</u> manner reflecting an expanded consciousness and universal connection. We are able to map our life, our behavior and purpose with greater sensitivity. We can act from a grater sense of moral purpose which is respecting the right of all life to evolve in their agreements with the universe. We work to serve others, as well as the common good, since all are connected, serving others, nourishes ourselves as well. We raise the spiritual evolution of the synchronicity field which is in harmony with the evolutionary direction of the universe. It is the never ending journey and search for evolutionary offerings and agreements for a profound and intimate love affair with the universe. It is a search for an orgasmic connection to an ever changing universe. That is the destination of an ephiphamonious journey, and it feels good too.

We embark upon an orgasmic connection to an ever changing universe.

It never stops until it stops, and even then it doesn't stop.

If you think you fully understand all of the above sayings, think again.

EPIPHAMONIOUS GLOSSARY

Epiphany; A sudden spiritual insight or overwhelming clarity of under-standing.

Epiph-anik; An epiphamonious follower.

Epipha-phermone; A fragrance reaching into one's innermost being.

Epic-epiphany; An exaggerated insight into one's personal universe.

Pickey-epiphany; A self critical insight to awaken one's self.

Epiphanon; A Shakespearian lurking epiphany.

Epipha-yawn; A tired epiphany.

Epipha-shtick; A humorous story which awakens one.

Epipha-moan; A response to an insightful pun.

Epipha-unanimous; A full agreement to a shared insight.

Epipha-nanny; A spiritual childrens caretaker.

Epiphony; A misleading insight.

Epup-aphfil; An insight in its infancy.

ABOUT THE AUTHOR

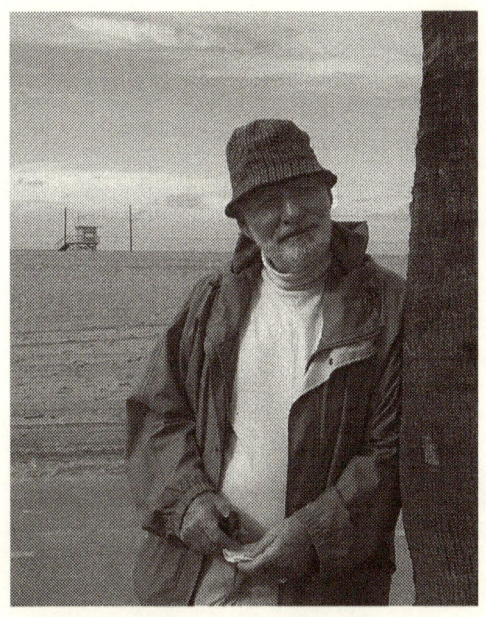

Photo by Eric Weinstein

Dr. Bob has been on his own journey of "not knowing who he is" exploring areas of homeopathy, holistic health, eastern healing arts and medicine, western psychotherapy, orthomolecular medicine, iridology, yoga and meditation, to name a few destinations visited. Receiving degrees from Boston Univ. Univ of Mich, and Univ of Southern Calif, he continued his journey as a professor, student, healer, and psychotherapist. He helped organize one of the first Holistic Health Centers in Southern California, and later became a director of a second. He has journeyed through several hospitals practicing as a medical and clinical social worker. He currently is exploring a writing career, and other ways to mangle the English language.

978-0-595-37934-7
0-595-37934-6